30-DAY FOOD-BASED SKIN HEALTH BOOK

Minimal Steps. Maximum Glow. All Skin Tones Welcome

STEPHANIE WILLIAMS, MBA

For permission requests, please contact:

Booked & Branded Publishing

www.bookedandbrandedpublishing.com

ISBN: 978-1-969369-26-1

Cover design, interior layout, and publishing by Booked & Branded Publishing.

Printed in the United States of America.

Disclaimer

This book is for educational purposes only. It is not intended as legal, financial, or credit repair advice. While the strategies shared are based on the author's personal experience and research, results may vary depending on individual circumstances. Readers are encouraged to seek guidance from qualified financial professionals before making credit or financial decisions. The author and publisher disclaim any liability for any loss or damage resulting from the use of this information.

For permission requests, get in touch with the publisher: Booked and Branded Publishing

Dedication

To anyone who has ever stared at their reflection and wondered if their skin could look brighter, feel smoother, or glow stronger — this book is for you. You deserve skin that reflects your inner strength, health, and confidence.

About the Author

Stephanie Williams, MBA — Strategic Business Consultant, author, and builder of beauty, brains, and business.

Stephanie is a visionary entrepreneur, and publishing powerhouse who helps others shine from the inside out. With an MBA from the Jack Welch Management Institute (perfect GPA, with a concentration in entrepreneurship) and years of experience at Verizon and Verizon Connect, she has developed expertise in corporate strategy and sales before building her own brand.

Her personal journey inspired her to write Blow Up Skincare and the 30-Day Food-Based Skin Health Book, uniting topical care with food-based strategies. Through Booked & Branded Publishing, she helps clients transform ideas into polished, profitable books and digital products.

When she isn't building brands and books, Stephanie curates wellness routines, empowers entrepreneurs, and designs a life where hustle meets strategy.

Table of Contents

Introduction

The Secret to Radiance from Within

Every woman desires luminous skin, but true radiance is more than creams, serums, or treatments. It begins much deeper—within the very cells of your body. The glow that turns heads and inspires confidence does not come from surface solutions. It comes from the food you choose, the rituals you practice, and the consistency you bring to your lifestyle.

In a world filled with promises of instant beauty, this book offers something more powerful: a path to lasting radiance. Here, you will discover how hydration, vitamins, minerals, healthy fats, probiotics, and superfoods work together to transform not only your skin but also your energy, mood, and presence.

This is not a diet book. It is a guide to building a legacy of beauty through nourishment. Every chapter has given you depth, insight, and strategies that feel both practical and luxurious. You will learn how to troubleshoot common skin concerns through nutrition, how to elevate your meals into rituals of elegance, and how to create a 30-Day Glow Challenge that resets and renews your body from the inside out.

Glow is not something you chase. It is something you create daily, through intentional choices. When you embrace this journey, your reflection changes, your confidence grows, and the way the world experiences you transform.

By the time you reach the final chapter, you will hold in your hands not just knowledge but a lifestyle plan—one that will keep your skin luminous, your body energized, and your spirit strong for years to come.

Welcome to your glow journey. Let this be the moment you stop seeking quick fixes and start building a beauty legacy that time cannot take away.

A Journey We Take Together

Think of this as a conversation, not a lecture. You'll get simple rituals, elegant recipes, and a 30-Day Food Glow Challenge that builds momentum one week at a time—hydration, renewal, balance, and antioxidant power—so you can see and feel changes quickly and sustainably.

Bring curiosity, not perfection. Consistency—more than intensity—wins the glow game.

Chapter 1

Why Food Matters for Your Skin

Your skin is not just your body's covering; it is a living organ that reflects everything you consume, think, and do. It is the canvas on which your habits, your nourishment, and your overall health are painted. If you want that canvas to radiate strength, vitality, and youthfulness, you cannot rely on surface treatments alone — you must nourish it from the inside out.

For years, the beauty industry has been driven by topical promises: a cream that erases wrinkles overnight. This serum delivers instant glow — a treatment that tightens skin in a single session. But no matter how advanced, topical care only treats the outermost layers of the skin. Nutrition works at the deepest level — fueling cells, supporting collagen production, and repairing damage long before it becomes visible.

Food vs. Topicals: The Two Pillars of Radiance

Think of food and skincare as partners in luxury living. Skincare products are like couture garments — they elevate your appearance. Food, however, is the tailoring of your body — invisible at first, but the foundation of everything others see.

- **Topicals are temporary.** They sit on the surface, offering a polished finish.
- **Food is permanent.** It transforms the skin from the inside, creating a glow that no makeup can replicate.

The two together form an unbeatable combination — the true secret behind ageless beauty.

The Science of Skin Nutrition

Your skin is constructed from proteins, lipids, water, and micronutrients. Everything you eat either strengthens this structure or weakens it.

- Proteins fuel collagen and elastin production — the very fibers that keep your face lifted and youthful.
- Healthy fats create the skin's lipid barrier, locking in moisture and giving you that supple, dewy finish.
- Antioxidants act as bodyguards, shielding cells from pollution, UV, and stress.
- Minerals ensure oxygen delivery, regulate oil production, and keep the skin resilient.

Every bite is building you up or breaking you down.

How Lifestyle Choices Appear on the Skin

Your skin is the ultimate truth-teller. Poor choices cannot be hidden for long.

- One night of poor sleep results in puffy eyes, pale skin, and a sluggish tone.
- Weeks of fast food led to breakouts, uneven texture, and fine lines.
- With consistent hydration, whole foods, and vitamins - skin glows without makeup.

Skin mirrors your internal world. Breakouts may appear if your digestion is sluggish. If your liver is overworked, dullness sets in. If your hormones are imbalanced, you may notice oiliness or dryness. Once you look at skin as a messenger instead of a problem, you unlock the key to long-term beauty.

The Luxury of Eating for Glow

Luxury isn't just designer handbags or spa days; it's the quiet discipline of daily choices that compound. Eating for your skin is a luxury act because it requires awareness, intention, and consistency.

- **Morning Rituals:** To detoxify and awaken digestion, begin with warm lemon water. This minor act brightens skin over time like a natural glow elixir.
- **Colorful Plates:** Think of your meals as palettes — reds from berries, greens from kale, yellows from turmeric. Each color is a different antioxidant working for your beauty.
- **Smart Snacking:** Swap empty calories for radiance-boosting foods: almonds instead of chips, dark chocolate instead of candy, sparkling water with lime instead of soda.

The elite don't just eat for energy; they eat for longevity, vibrancy, and beauty. You deserve the same standards.

Food + Skincare: The Glow Multiplier

Food doesn't replace your creams, and creams don't replace your meals. Together, they enhance one another.

- A Vitamin C serum delivers brightness — but paired with citrus, kiwi, and peppers in your diet, the glow is amplified tenfold.
- A hyaluronic acid moisturizer hydrates the skin — but only if your body is also hydrated with water, fruits, and electrolytes.
- Collagen powders improve firmness — but only if combined with protein-rich meals and Vitamin C for absorption.

This dual-care method is how you transition from temporary results to a lasting, glowing legacy.

Building a Skin-Nourishing Mindset

Food is not punishment, and skincare is not vanity. Both are investments. Think of your plate as your most powerful beauty treatment.

Shift your perspective with these mindset upgrades:

- From deprivation - to nourishment. Don't ask, "What do I have to give up?" Instead, ask, "What can I add that supports my glow?"
- From quick fixes - to lifestyle upgrades. A single green smoothie won't change your skin — but 30 days of nutrient-rich eating will.
- From cost - to value. A bag of chips costs money and steals radiance. A handful of walnuts costs money and builds collagen. Which is the better investment?

Case Study: Two Women, Two Outcomes

- Clara, 42, relied only on creams. She spent thousands yearly on facials, serums, and treatments. Her skin looked good under makeup but tired without it.
- Diana, 42, combined skincare with intentional nutrition. She hydrated daily, added antioxidants at each meal, and balanced proteins with healthy fats.

Her skin looked radiant, even without makeup, and she required fewer cosmetic products.

The difference? Diana treated food as her skincare. Clara treated skincare as her only solution. One invested on the surface; the other invested from the foundation up.

Key Takeaway

Your glow is not luck. It is a strategy. Serums polish. Food transforms. If you want to build beauty that lasts decades, not days, it begins with the choices on your plate.

CHAPTER 2

Hydration & Detox Basics

If food is the foundation of healthy skin, hydration is the lifeblood that keeps that foundation strong. Your skin comprises almost 64% water, which is crucial for its functions like cell renewal, elasticity, repair, and natural detoxification. When hydration is lacking, the skin speaks: fine lines appear deeper, flakiness takes over, and the complexion looks tired and aged.

Glowing skin is not just about what you put on your face; it begins with what you pour into your glass.

Why Hydration Matters for Radiance

Think of water as your skin's internal moisturizer. While creams and oils lock moisture into the outer layer, water circulates through every cell, delivering nutrients and flushing out toxins.

- **Plumpness:** Hydrated skin cells are full and bouncy, softening fine lines.

- **Clarity:** Water helps transport nutrients to the skin and supports detoxification, preventing dullness.
- **Healing:** Proper hydration speeds up wound healing, reduces inflammation, and strengthens your skin barrier.
- **Protection:** Well-hydrated skin is less sensitive to environmental stressors like pollution, sun, and dry air.

Without enough hydration, even the most expensive serums cannot deliver their promise.

How Much Water Do You Need?

There's no one-size-fits-all, but here is a practical guideline:

- Drink at least half your body weight in ounces of water daily.
- Add an extra 12—18 ounces if you're exercising, sweating, or living in tropical climates.

For example, a 150-pound woman should aim for about 75 ounces daily, increasing if she works out or spends time outdoors.

Luxury Tip: Don't just count glasses, curate your hydration. Choose infused waters, sparkling mineral water, or coconut water to make hydration feel like an indulgence rather than a chore.

Beyond Water: The Role of Electrolytes

Hydration is not just about how much water you drink; it's about how much water your cells can hold. This is where electrolytes come in.

- **Sodium and potassium** help balance fluids inside and outside cells.
- **Magnesium** supports over 300 enzymatic processes, including those that regulate hydration.
- **Calcium** plays a key role in skin cell renewal and repair.

Pro Tip: Add a pinch of sea salt, a squeeze of citrus, or drink natural coconut water to help water stay inside your cells instead of passing straight through.

Detox-Supporting Foods

Your skin thrives when your body eliminates waste. When detoxification slows, breakouts, puffiness, and uneven tone can appear. Hydration is the ultimate detoxifier, but you can strengthen the effect with cleansing foods:

- **Cucumbers:** cooling, water-rich, and packed with silica for skin elasticity.
- **Lemon:** Supports liver detox pathways and brightens skin tone.
- **Leafy greens:** Fuel your body with chlorophyll, nature's cleanser.

- **Watermelon:** Hydrates while delivering antioxidants like lycopene.

Luxury Ritual: Start mornings with warm lemon water, add cucumber slices to your daily water pitcher, and finish the evening with a calming herbal tea like dandelion or chamomile to support overnight detox.

Hydration Habits of the Radiant

It's not just about drinking more water; it's about building habits that make hydration second nature.

- **The 1:1 Rule:** For every cup of coffee or alcohol, drink one glass of water.
- **Front-load Hydration:** Drink most of your water before 6 p.m. to avoid restless sleep.
- **Elegant Vessels:** Use a beautiful glass or water bottle. When hydration feels luxurious, you'll want more.
- **Hydrating Foods:** Remember, food counts too. Soups, fruits, vegetables, and smoothies contribute to your daily intake.

Hydration and Aging

As we age, our skin loses moisture more quickly. This makes hydration not just a daily habit but a lifelong commitment to aging with elegance. A hydrated woman looks fresher, calmer, and more confident. Her glow speaks of discipline and care.

Case in Point: Imagine two women at 50. One drinks water and relies on creams. The other prioritizes hydration daily with infused water, teas, and water-rich foods. The second woman's skin radiates vitality and elasticity, while the first struggles with dryness and visible lines. The difference isn't luck — it's lifestyle.

Key Takeaway

Hydration is the most luxurious, non-negotiable step in your glow plan. Pair water with electrolytes and detoxifying foods, and treat hydration like a beauty ritual — not a task. Remember: skincare sits on the surface, but hydration builds beauty at the cellular level.

Chapter 3

Vitamin C — The Glow Booster

If hydration is the foundation of radiant skin, Vitamin C is the spark that ignites the glow. Known as the queen of radiance, Vitamin C does more than brighten the surface. It works deep within the skin to stimulate collagen, reduce pigmentation, and protect against environmental stressors. This single nutrient carries the power to transform dull, uneven complexions into luminous, youthful skin.

Why Vitamin C is Essential for Skin Health

Vitamin C is one of the most potent antioxidants in nature.

It plays multiple roles in protecting and renewing the skin because:

- It stimulates collagen production, keeping skin firm, lifted, and youthful.

- It helps fade hyperpigmentation and dark spots, creating an even tone.
- It neutralizes free radicals caused by pollution, sun exposure, and stress.
- It enhances the skin's ability to repair itself, reducing inflammation and redness.

Without adequate Vitamin C, skin appears tired, sags more quickly, and heals more slowly. With it, you unlock the true glow your skin shows.

Food as Your Vitamin C Serum

While serums deliver Vitamin C, consuming it through food brings results at the cellular level. When you nourish your body with Vitamin C-rich foods, you are feeding your skin from within. The effect is longer-lasting and more powerful than any cream alone.

Excellent food sources include:

- Citrus fruits such as oranges, lemons, and grapefruits.
- Bright produce such as kiwi, strawberries, and papayas.
- Vegetables such as bell peppers, kale, and broccoli.

Eating a rainbow of Vitamin C-rich foods ensures your body has a steady supply for collagen production and daily protection.

The Glow-Boosting Rituals of Vitamin C

Vitamin C is not just about occasional consumption. It is about weaving it into your lifestyle so your skin is fueled.

Here are practices to elevate your daily glow:

- Begin the morning with warm lemon water or fresh citrus juice to awaken digestion and deliver an antioxidant boost.
- Add colorful peppers, tomatoes, and leafy greens to your lunch and dinner for steady collagen support.
- Snack on strawberries or kiwi in the afternoon for a natural, skin-brightening lift.
- Pair Vitamin C foods with iron-rich meals such as spinach or lentils to improve absorption and maximize energy.

By making these habits consistent, your skin will look more vibrant week after week.

Vitamin C and Collagen: Your Skin's Firmness Factor

One of the most important roles of Vitamin C is its direct involvement in collagen synthesis. Collagen is the structural protein that keeps your skin firm and plump. Without Vitamin C, collagen fibers weaken, leading to sagging and wrinkles. With it, your skin becomes more elastic, more youthful, and more resilient.

Think of Vitamin C as the architect that directs collagen production. Without the architect, the builders cannot complete their work.

Vitamin C as Your Skin's Bodyguard

Every day, your skin faces invisible threats: pollution in the air, ultraviolet rays from the sun, and internal stress that triggers inflammation. These stressors create free radicals, unstable molecules that damage skin cells and speed up aging.

Vitamin C acts as a shield. By neutralizing free radicals before they cause harm, it slows the visible signs of aging and preserves your glow. Therefore, women who consume Vitamin C often appear years younger than their actual age.

Case Study: The Radiance Difference

Consider two women in their thirties. One has a diet heavy in processed foods and little fresh produce. Her skin appears tired, with uneven tone and fine lines beginning to surface. The other includes Vitamin C at every meal, drinks citrus-infused water, and snacks on colorful fruits. Her skin appears fresh, radiant, and more youthful than her years.

The difference lies not in genetics alone but in daily nourishment. Radiance is not accidental. It is intentional.

Luxury Living with Vitamin C

True luxury is not about quick fixes but about building habits that make beauty inevitable. Incorporating Vitamin C-rich foods into elegant rituals transforms health into a lifestyle of radiance. Imagine hosting a brunch with a vibrant citrus salad, enjoying green tea with lemon in the afternoon, or finishing dinner with a bowl of fresh berries. These small yet intentional acts create a sense of indulgence while working to maintain your skin's youthfulness.

Key Takeaway

Vitamin C is not a vitamin. It is the glow booster, the collagen activator, and the protector that your skin cannot live without. By weaving Vitamin C-rich foods into your life, you transform not only your complexion but also your energy, your confidence, and your presence. Your glow becomes a signature of discipline, care, and elegance.

CHAPTER 4

Vitamin A — Renewal from Within

Every radiant complexion begins with renewal. The skin you see today is not the same skin you had yesterday; it is shedding old cells and creating new ones. At the center of this renewal process is Vitamin A. Known as the nutrient of transformation, Vitamin A helps your skin regenerate, unclogs pores, smooths texture, and restores the vibrancy that time and stress often steal away.

Without Vitamin A, skin renewal slows. Cells build up on the surface, leading to roughness, clogged pores, and dullness. With Vitamin A, renewal is constant, revealing fresh, and youthful skin.

The Science of Renewal: Why Vitamin A Matters

Vitamin A is essential for maintaining healthy skin because it

- Stimulates cell turnover, helping to replace old, dull cells with fresh ones.
- Regulates oil production, keeping pores clear and reducing the risk of acne.
- Supports the skin's natural healing process, which minimizes scarring and uneven texture.
- Enhances collagen production, improving skin firmness and elasticity.

Therefore, dermatologists often refer to Vitamin A as a "gold-standard" nutrient for both beauty and longevity.

Beta-Carotene vs. Retinol: Two Powerful Forms

Vitamin A comes in two primary forms, each with its own unique contribution to your glow.

- Beta-carotene (Plant-Based Precursor): found in orange and green vegetables such as sweet potatoes, carrots, and spinach. Your body converts beta-carotene into Vitamin A as needed, making it a safe and steady source.
- Retinol (Animal-Based Active Form): Found in eggs, dairy, and liver. This form is already active, making it efficient at fueling skin renewal.

Including both forms in your diet ensures your body always has the tools it needs for repair and radiance.

Pairing Vitamin A with Healthy Fats

Vitamin A is fat-soluble, meaning it requires dietary fat for effective absorption. Without fat, much of it passes through the body without being used. Therefore, pairing Vitamin A foods with healthy fats makes all the difference.

- Sweet potatoes with a drizzle of olive oil.
- Spinach sautéed in avocado oil.
- Carrots dipped in hummus or nut butter.
- Eggs cooked with a side of avocado.

These simple combinations turn ordinary meals into powerful skin-renewing therapies.

Vitamin A and Acne Healing

One of Vitamin A's most remarkable benefits is its ability to regulate oil production and prevent clogged pores. Many prescription acne treatments are derivatives of Vitamin A, proving its power to transform troubled skin.

By incorporating natural sources into your diet, you can support clearer, calmer skin without harsh treatments. For those who struggle with breakouts, Vitamin A becomes not just a nutrient but a daily defense.

Vitamin A for Anti-Aging and Texture

As we age, cell turnover slows. Therefore, skin looks rougher, fine lines deepen, and overall radiance fades. Vitamin A speeds up the skin's renewal cycle, allowing it to appear younger and smoother.

Regular intake of Vitamin A-rich foods, combined with topical support if desired, helps maintain a refined texture and a soft glow that reflects youth and vitality.

The Luxury Ritual of Renewal

Incorporating Vitamin A into your lifestyle can feel indulgent and elegant. Imagine starting your day with a vibrant smoothie made from carrots, mango, and spinach, rich in beta-carotene. Lunch might include a vibrant spinach salad topped with eggs and avocado. Dinner could feature roasted sweet potatoes with a drizzle of olive oil.

Each meal is both nourishment and luxury, not just filling your plate but renewing your skin with every bite.

Case Study: The Clear Skin Advantage

Consider two men in their twenties. Both struggled with oily, acne-prone skin. One continued with a diet heavy in processed snacks, fried foods, and sugary drinks. His skin remained inflamed and prone to breakouts. The other began introducing Vitamin A-rich foods, pairing them with healthy fats daily. Within weeks, his breakouts calmed, his pores appeared smaller, and his skin tone looked clearer.

The transformation was not luck, but a deliberate strategy. Consistency with Vitamin A created the foundation for long-term clarity and confidence.

Key Takeaway

Vitamin A is the nutrient of renewal. It fuels cell turnover, unclogs pores, smooths texture, and restores youthful radiance. By including both beta-carotene and retinol sources in your diet and pairing them with healthy fats, you activate the natural renewal cycle your skin craves. Renewal is not accidental; it results from intentional nourishment.

CHAPTER 5

Vitamin E — Protection and Repair

Every radiant complexion needs both strength and defense. While Vitamin C brightens and Vitamin A renews, Vitamin E protects. Known as the skin's shield, Vitamin E is one of the most potent antioxidants available, guarding your complexion from environmental damage, repairing tissues at the cellular level, and slowing the visible signs of aging.

When your body is low in Vitamin E, skin can appear fragile, dull, and more vulnerable to sun damage. With it, you gain a natural barrier of resilience, leaving your skin smooth, nourished, and glowing with confidence.

Why Vitamin E is Called the Skin's Bodyguard

Vitamin E is a fat-soluble nutrient that integrates into cell membranes, strengthening them from within. This characteristic makes it a powerful protector against damage caused by ultraviolet rays, pollution, and oxidative stress.

- It prevents free radicals from breaking down collagen and elastin.
- It reduces inflammation, calming irritated and sensitive skin.
- It speeds up tissue repair, minimizing scars and rough patches.
- It locks in moisture, keeping skin soft.

Every cell in your skin benefits from Vitamin E, which is why it is often called your body's first line of defense against premature aging.

Food Sources of Vitamin E

Nature offers Vitamin E in a variety of nutrient-dense foods. Adding them to your diet daily is an effortless way to strengthen and protect your glow.

- Almonds, hazelnuts, and sunflower seeds.
- Avocados and olives.
- Plant oils such as sunflower, wheat germ, and extra virgin olive oil.
- Dark leafy greens such as spinach and Swiss chard.

Luxury Tip: Keep a small container of raw almonds or hazelnuts in your bag. It is not only an elegant snack but also a consistent way to provide your skin with protective Vitamin E throughout the day.

Vitamin E and Sun Protection

While sunscreen is essential for guarding against UV damage, Vitamin E offers an internal layer of protection. Studies show that individuals with higher Vitamin E levels experience less oxidative damage from sun exposure.

This does not mean Vitamin E replaces sunscreen, but it reinforces your defense system, reducing the long-term risk of sunspots, wrinkles, and uneven pigmentation.

Vitamin E and Scar Healing

One of Vitamin E's most notable roles is in supporting wound healing and reducing the appearance of scars. By nourishing new cells and reducing inflammation, it helps skin recover more smoothly. From acne marks to minor cuts, a diet rich in Vitamin E supports the natural repair process.

Moisture and Resilience from Within

Because Vitamin E strengthens the skin's lipid barrier, it helps lock in hydration. This is especially important as skin matures and natural oil production decreases. Adequate Vitamin E ensures that moisture remains where it belongs — inside your cells.

Women who consume Vitamin E often notice fewer dry patches and a smoother, more even texture, even without heavy creams.

Luxury Rituals with Vitamin E

Adding Vitamin E to your lifestyle can be both simple and elegant.

- Begin the day with a smoothie blended with spinach, avocado, and sunflower seeds.
- Drizzle extra virgin olive oil over roasted vegetables or salads for a dose of antioxidants.
- End the evening with a small piece of dark chocolate paired with almonds, combining indulgence with nourishment.

Each choice becomes a ritual of protection, building beauty from the inside out.

Case Study: Protection vs. Vulnerability

Two women in their forties both loved spending time outdoors. One relied only on sunscreen for protection, while the other paired sunscreen with a diet rich in Vitamin E from nuts, seeds, and avocados. Years later, the first struggled with fine lines, sunspots, and uneven tone. The second, though the same age, maintained smoother skin, fewer dark patches, and a stronger overall glow.

The difference was not just in what they applied but in what they consumed. Vitamin E provided a level of internal repair and protection that creams alone could not achieve.

Key Takeaway

Vitamin E is the guardian of your glow. By protecting against environmental damage, reducing inflammation, locking in moisture, and speeding up repair, it ensures that your skin not only looks radiant but remains resilient. Incorporating Vitamin E-rich foods into your daily diet is one of the most powerful long-term investments you can make in your beauty. Protection is not optional. It is the key to lasting radiance.

CHAPTER 6

Vitamin K — Brightness and Balance

Every radiant face has one thing in common: a sense of balance. True glow is not just about brightness or hydration, but about the evenness of tone and the calmness of the complexion. This is where Vitamin K steps in. Often overlooked in the world of beauty, Vitamin K is the quiet force that strengthens capillaries, reduces dark circles, calms redness, and promotes a more even skin appearance. It is the nutrient that ensures your glow looks smooth, refined, and balanced.

Without Vitamin K, blood vessels become more fragile, leading to visible redness, uneven skin tone, and shadows under the eyes. With it, your complexion looks brighter, calmer, and more refreshed.

Why Vitamin K is Essential for Radiance

Vitamin K supports circulation and strengthens blood vessels beneath the skin's surface. Poor circulation can cause blood to gather, resulting in dark under-eye circles, uneven skin tone, and color changes. By reinforcing this delicate system, Vitamin K helps skin look healthier and more even.

Its key benefits include:

- Brightens dark under-eye circles.
- Reducing redness from broken capillaries or irritation.
- Supporting skin healing after blemishes or minor bruising.
- Enhances the overall balance of skin tone.

Food Sources of Vitamin K

Vitamin K is abundant in many green vegetables and herbs. By including these in your meals, you provide your skin with a steady supply of balance-building nutrients.

- Spinach, kale, and Swiss chard.
- Broccoli, Brussels sprouts, and green beans.
- Fresh herbs such as parsley, basil, and cilantro.
- Fermented foods like natto, which contain a powerful form of Vitamin K.

Luxury Tip: Create vibrant meals that look as beautiful as they taste. A kale and spinach salad with olive oil and a sprinkle of fresh parsley is not only nourishing but elegant, making your dining experience feel indulgent while protecting your glow.

Vitamin K and Dark Circles

Few things make a face look more tired than dark circles. While lack of sleep and genetics play a role, weak capillaries beneath the eyes are often the hidden cause. Vitamin K strengthens these tiny vessels, reducing the pooling of blood that causes shadowing.

Regular intake of Vitamin K-rich foods, along with proper hydration, can help the under-eye area appear lighter, fresher, and more youthful.

Vitamin K and Redness

If you struggle with redness or visible capillaries on the cheeks and nose, Vitamin K offers support by calming inflammation and strengthening blood vessel walls. Therefore, many topical creams designed for sensitive or redness-prone skin include Vitamin K. By combining external and internal use, you reinforce results both at the surface and within the skin.

Healing Power of Vitamin K

Vitamin K also plays a role in the body's natural healing process. When the skin is injured, whether from acne blemishes or minor cuts, Vitamin K supports clotting and tissue repair. This leads to smoother healing, fewer marks, and a more even complexion.

Luxury Rituals with Vitamin K

Adding Vitamin K to your lifestyle can feel elegant and effortless.

- Begin the day with a green smoothie made of spinach, parsley, and pineapple.
- Enjoy a lunch of roasted Brussels sprouts with olive oil.
- Add chopped fresh herbs to your evening dishes for both flavor and radiance.
- Consider a calming evening tea made with nettle or parsley leaves to support circulation.

These rituals not only provide balance but also elevate your dining into beauty care.

Case Study: the Balanced Glow

Imagine two women in their late thirties. Both lead busy lives and often look tired. One neglects leafy greens and eats herbs or vegetables. Her skin shows more redness, her under-eye circles darken, and her tone appears uneven. The other prioritizes Vitamin K-rich meals, blending smoothies, adding greens to every plate, and enjoying fresh herbs daily. Her complexion appears calm, bright, and balanced. She looks rested even on long days.

The difference is not luck but nourishment. Vitamin K became her secret to sustained radiance.

Key Takeaway

Vitamin K is the nutrient of balance. By strengthening capillaries, reducing dark circles, calming redness, and supporting healing, it ensures that your glow looks even and refined. Through consistent consumption of Vitamin K-rich foods, you cultivate not just brightness but harmony in your complexion. Radiance is not only about light; it is also about balance, and Vitamin K provides that.

Chapter 7

B Vitamins — Energy and Elasticity

When people think of glowing skin, they often focus on surface treatments or single miracle nutrients. Yet, behind the scenes, a family of vitamins works to energize, repair, and protect your skin. This is the family of B Vitamins. These essential nutrients are not just about beauty; they are about vitality. When your body has enough B Vitamins, your skin reflects energy, resilience, and elasticity. When it does not, the first signs often appear on your face as dullness, dryness, or premature fine lines.

The beauty of B Vitamins lies in their collective power. They do not work in isolation. Instead, they function as a team, supporting metabolism, stress response, and cell renewal. Together, they create a foundation where both energy and beauty thrive

The Role of B Vitamins in Skin Health

Each B Vitamin has its own unique role, but all contribute to glow and elasticity.

- Vitamin B12 helps prevent dryness and supports oxygen delivery to skin cells. Without it, skin often looks pale, tired, and fragile.
- Vitamin B3 (niacin) improves circulation and strengthens the skin barrier, making skin more elastic. It is also known for its calming effect on inflammation.
- Folate (Vitamin B9) repairs tissue and assists in new cell formation, ensuring that your complexion stays fresh and youthful.

By combining these and other B Vitamins, you give your skin the energy it needs to resist stress-driven dullness.

Energy for Radiance

Skin that glows always begins with energy at the cellular level. B Vitamins are vital in converting the food you eat into usable energy. When your body functions, your skin receives the oxygen and nutrients it needs to stay vibrant.

A lack of B Vitamins often manifests as fatigue, which the skin reflects through dullness, a lack of color, and slower healing. By maintaining a steady intake of B Vitamins, you can support the vitality that makes your skin radiant from the inside.

B Vitamins and Stress

Modern life is filled with stress, and the body's stress response can drain reserves of B Vitamins. Stress not only exhausts energy but also weakens the skin barrier, leading to irritation and breakouts. Ensuring that your body has adequate B Vitamins acts like a buffer against these effects, helping your skin remain calm, elastic, and balanced even in challenging seasons.

Food Sources of B Vitamins

Fortunately, B Vitamins are abundant in a wide variety of whole foods.

- Eggs and fish provide vitamin B12.
- Legumes, such as lentils and chickpeas, are rich in folate.
- Mushrooms, seeds, and poultry offer multiple B Vitamins, including niacin.
- Whole grains contribute to the overall B complex that supports metabolism.

Luxury Tip: Create meals that combine multiple sources of B Vitamins. A breakfast of scrambled eggs with sautéed mushrooms or a dinner of salmon with lentils offers not only nourishment but also elegance, giving your body the complete support it needs.

The Elasticity Connection

Elasticity is the ability of skin to stretch and return to its natural shape. With age and stress, elasticity decreases, leading to sagging and fine lines. Niacin, folate, and other B Vitamins help strengthen the skin barrier and support collagen, keeping the skin supple and firm. Consistency is key. The more often you nourish your body with B Vitamins, the longer your skin maintains its youthful bounce.

Luxury Rituals with B Vitamins

Incorporating B Vitamins can be part of your daily rituals.

- Begin your day with a protein-rich breakfast of eggs, whole grains, and fresh vegetables.
- Choose a midday snack of roasted chickpeas or hummus with vegetables.
- Enjoy a dinner of grilled fish paired with a lentil or quinoa salad.
- For an elegant touch, include shiitake mushrooms in stir-fries or soups to provide both flavor and nourishment.

These rituals transform simple meals into a refined practice of energy and beauty care.

Case Study: Energy Restored, Glow Renewed

Consider two professionals in their early forties. Both lead stressful lives with long working hours. One often skips meals or relies on processed snacks, leaving her skin looking fatigued, pale, and lined. The other makes B Vitamin-rich foods a priority, keeping boiled eggs, lentils, and fresh vegetables as part of her daily routine. Over time, her skin looks fresh, smooth, and elastic, reflecting the vitality within her body.

The difference lies in energy management. By fueling the body with B Vitamins, she not only preserved her health but also achieved visible radiance.

Key Takeaway

B Vitamins are the hidden architects of energy and elasticity. They prevent dryness, repair tissue, improve circulation, and protect against stress-driven dullness. By consuming foods rich in the B family, you give your skin the resilience and vitality it needs to remain youthful. Radiance is not only about brightness but also about energy and strength, and B Vitamins deliver both.

Chapter 8

Minerals that Matter

If vitamins are the sparks that ignite radiance, minerals are the steady pillars that sustain it. They are the quiet yet essential elements that regulate the body's internal systems and influence the health of your skin. Without minerals, even the best diet and skincare routine falls short. With them, your skin gains strength, balance, and vitality that endures.

Why Minerals are Essential for Skin Health

Minerals act as cofactors in countless biological reactions. They support oxygen delivery, regulate oil production, and defend against oxidative stress. Unlike some vitamins, the body cannot produce minerals on its own. They must be consumed daily through food. The quality of your glow is therefore linked to the minerals on your plate.

Zinc: The Balancer of Breakouts

Zinc is one of the most powerful minerals for skin health. It regulates oil production, reduces inflammation, and speeds up wound healing. This makes it important for those prone to acne or breakouts.

Foods rich in zinc include oysters, pumpkin seeds, and chickpeas.

Luxury Tip: A refined way to enjoy zinc is through a seafood dinner featuring oysters or grilled salmon paired with pumpkin seed garnish. It transforms nourishment into indulgence.

Selenium: The Protector of Elasticity

Selenium works with Vitamin E to protect the skin against oxidative stress and UV damage. It plays a vital role in preserving elasticity and slowing premature aging.

Rich food sources include Brazil nuts, tuna, and whole grains. Even a single Brazil nut a day can provide enough selenium to support your overall well-being and radiance.

Iron: The Oxygen Carrier

Iron ensures that oxygen is delivered to every cell, including those in the skin. When iron is lacking, the result is pale, dull, and tired-looking skin. Adequate iron keeps skin vibrant, energized, and luminous.

Iron is found in spinach, lentils, and lean meats. Pairing iron-rich foods with Vitamin C sources enhances absorption, making your meals both balanced and efficient.

Magnesium: The Stress Soother

Though often overlooked in skin conversations, magnesium is essential for regulating stress and calming inflammation. Stress depletes skin of nutrients and speeds up aging, but magnesium helps restore balance.

Sources include dark leafy greens, nuts, seeds, and whole grains. Ending the evening with magnesium-rich herbal tea or almonds is both soothing and beautifying.

Mineral Synergy: Working Together

Minerals do not act alone. Zinc works with Vitamin A to regulate oil production. Selenium pairs with Vitamin E to strengthen the skin's barrier. Iron depends on Vitamin C for absorption. This interconnectedness is why a varied diet rich in whole foods is more effective than relying on supplements.

Luxury Rituals with Minerals

You can design elegant meals and snacks that provide a spectrum of minerals.

- A breakfast of a spinach and mushroom omelet.

- A mid-morning handful of mixed nuts with a single Brazil nut.
- A dinner of grilled salmon with lentils and leafy greens.
- A dessert of dark chocolate paired with pumpkin seeds.

These rituals not only elevate your palate but also ensure consistent mineral support for your skin.

Case Study: Mineral Glow vs. Mineral Gap

Two men in their thirties followed very different diets. One relied on fast food, leaving him low in zinc, iron, and magnesium. His skin often looked oily, pale, and fatigued. The other consumed a variety of seafood, nuts, and vegetables rich in minerals. His skin remained firm, even-toned, and glowing.

The difference was not luck but mineral consistency. Beauty is built on the nutrients you consume, not occasionally.

Key Takeaway

Minerals are the unseen foundation of radiance. Zinc balances oil and heals blemishes, selenium preserves elasticity, iron fuels oxygen delivery, and magnesium calms stress. Together, they provide the stability your skin needs to thrive. Consistency is the secret. When minerals are part of your daily lifestyle, your glow becomes unshakable.

Chapter 9

Omega-3s and Healthy Fats

If hydration keeps your skin supple and vitamins brighten your complexion, healthy fats are the element that gives skin its luxurious softness and long-lasting moisture. Omega-3 fatty acids and other nourishing fats are the foundation of a radiant, youthful glow. They strengthen the skin barrier, calm inflammation, and create the luminous texture that no cream can achieve alone.

When the body lacks healthy fats, skin often becomes dry, inflamed, and prone to premature lines. When the body is nourished with omega-3s and supportive fats, skin appears plump, smooth, and vibrant.

Why Healthy Fats are Essential for Radiance

Fats are not the enemy. In fact, the right kinds of fats are among the most potent tools for glowing skin. They form part of the lipid barrier that keeps moisture locked into skin cells. Without them, water escapes, leading to dryness and roughness.

Healthy fats also reduce inflammation, a common cause of redness, acne, and irritation. By calming the skin at its foundation, omega-3s create balance, ensuring your glow is smooth and even.

Omega-3s: The Anti-Inflammatory Heroes

Omega-3 fatty acids are essential because the body cannot produce them on its own. They must be consumed through diet. Their benefits for the skin include:

- Strengthening the skin's natural barrier.
- Reducing redness and irritation caused by inflammation.
- Supporting collagen, helping to preserve firmness.
- Hydrating skin from within for a dewy texture.

Foods rich in omega-3 fatty acids include salmon, mackerel, sardines, walnuts, chia seeds, and flaxseeds.

Beyond Omega-3: Other Healthy Fats for Glow

While omega-3s are the star, other fats also contribute to radiance. Monounsaturated fats, found in avocados and olive oil, provide deep nourishment. Medium-chain triglycerides in coconut oil offer quick energy and moisture support.

Together, these fats ensure your glow is both sustained and balanced.

The Connection Between Fats and Aging

As we age, the skin's natural oil production decreases, leading to dryness and fine lines. By consuming healthy fats, you replenish what the body loses. Therefore, women who embrace healthy fats in their diets often maintain soft skin long after others notice dryness and sagging.

Luxury Rituals with Healthy Fats

Incorporating healthy fats into your meals can feel indulgent and refined.

- Begin the morning with chia seed pudding topped with walnuts and berries.
- Add avocado slices to salads or whole grain toast for a creamy, satisfying upgrade.
- Prepare salmon for dinner drizzled with olive oil and served with roasted vegetables.
- Enjoy a spoonful of flaxseeds stirred into smoothies for a subtle, nourishing boost.

Each ritual combines elegance with nourishment, making healthy fats a natural part of your beauty care.

Case Study: Dryness vs. Dewiness

Two women in their mid-thirties maintained very different eating habits. One avoided fats, believing they were unhealthy. Over time, her skin became dry, her fine lines deepened, and she struggled with uneven texture. The other embraced omega-3-rich meals, eating salmon, avocado, and chia seeds. Her skin remained soft, dewy, and resilient, reflecting years of consistent nourishment.

The difference was not genetics but perspective. Healthy fats became the investment that preserved her glow.

Key Takeaway

Omega-3s and healthy fats are the moisturizers your skin craves from within. They build resilience, reduce inflammation, and keep your complexion supple and luminous. By making healthy fats a daily habit, you choose a glow that lasts not for days but for decades. True beauty is not about avoiding fats. It is about choosing the right ones and embracing them as essential to your radiance.

CHAPTER 10

Probiotics and the Gut-Skin Connection

If the skin is the mirror of health, the gut is the foundation that shapes what you see. Over seventy percent of your immune system lives in the gut, and countless studies now confirm that gut balance influences skin clarity, brightness, and resilience. A calm, healthy digestive system translates to glowing skin, while imbalance often reveals itself through breakouts, inflammation, dullness, or premature aging.

When your gut is nourished, your skin radiates health. If not attended to, no cream can bring back its best appearance.

Why Gut Health Matters for Your Glow

The gut and skin are connected through what scientists call the gut-skin axis. This pathway links digestion, immunity, and inflammation to the complexion.

- A balanced gut reduces systemic inflammation, preventing redness and irritation on the skin.
- A healthy gut microbiome strengthens the skin barrier, reducing sensitivity.
- Digestive efficiency ensures that nutrients are absorbed, fueling cell renewal and repair.

When your gut is thriving, your skin does not just look better; it functions better.

Probiotics: The Skin's Allies

Probiotics are beneficial bacteria that live in your digestive system. They keep harmful bacteria under control and help create an internal environment that supports beauty from the inside out.

Food sources of probiotics include yogurt, kefir, kimchi, sauerkraut, miso, and kombucha. These foods replenish the microbiome and calm inflammation, resulting in clearer, more even-toned skin.

Luxury Tip: Elevate your daily probiotic habit by choosing artisanal yogurts, handcrafted kimchi, or specialty kombucha blends. When wellness feels indulgent, consistency becomes effortless.

Prebiotics: Feeding the Glow

Just as flowers need soil to thrive, probiotics need prebiotics to flourish. Prebiotics are fibers that feed healthy gut bacteria, allowing them to multiply and work more effectively.

Excellent prebiotic sources include bananas, garlic, onions, asparagus, and oats. When combined with probiotics, they create a powerful synergy known as synbiotics, which maximize gut health benefits.

For example, pairing yogurt with banana or kefir with oats turns a simple meal into a glow-enhancing ritual.

The Gut and Inflammation Connection

Many common skin conditions, such as acne, eczema, and rosacea, are linked to inflammation that begins in the gut. An imbalanced microbiome can leak toxins into the bloodstream, triggering immune responses that show up as redness, breakouts, or irritation. By restoring balance through probiotics and prebiotics, inflammation decreases, and skin calms.

Gut Health and Emotional Radiance

Your gut not only affects your physical health. It also influences your mood through the production of serotonin, the hormone often referred to as the "happiness chemical." When you feel balanced and calm, your skin reflects that emotional wellness. Therefore, many people who improve gut health notice not only better skin but also increased confidence and a sense of inner glow.

Luxury Rituals with Probiotics and Prebiotics

Making gut health a daily ritual is both practical and refined.

- Begin the morning with a bowl of yogurt topped with bananas and chia seeds.
- Enjoy a midday snack of apple slices paired with almond butter and a sprinkle of oats.
- Add a side of kimchi or sauerkraut to lunch or dinner for both flavor and balance.
- Sip a glass of kombucha in the afternoon as an elegant alternative to soda.

Each choice is a graceful investment in both gut balance and skin brilliance.

Case Study: Clear Skin from Within

Consider two young women with similar lifestyles. Both struggled with acne in their early twenties. One relied only on topical treatments, layering creams and cleansers, but ignored her gut health. Her breakouts continued to return—the other incorporated probiotics and prebiotics daily, restoring her gut balance. Within months, her skin cleared, her tone evened out, and her confidence grew.

The transformation was not magic, but a balance of the microbiome. Skin healed because the gut healed first.

Key Takeaway

Your gut and skin are in constant conversation. Probiotics replenish the balance, prebiotics fuel the process, and together they create a harmony that shows on your face. By treating gut care as part of your beauty regimen, you not only build healthier digestion but also achieve lasting radiance. Glow begins in the gut, and nurturing it is one of the most powerful choices you can make for lifelong beauty.

CHAPTER 11

Collagen and Protein Power

When people speak of youthful skin, they are speaking about collagen. Collagen is a protein that provides structure, firmness, and elasticity. It is the framework that holds your skin in place, keeping it smooth and lifted. Without collagen, skin sags, lines deepen, and the bounce of youth fades.

Protein is the foundation of collagen production. Every strand of collagen is built from amino acids that come from the food you eat. If your diet is low in protein, your body cannot build or repair collagen, no matter how many creams you apply. When you pair protein with the right boosters, you create the ultimate formula for long-lasting firmness and radiance.

Why Collagen is the Key to Youthful Skin

Collagen makes up eighty percent of the skin's structure. It gives your face its shape and resilience. With age, collagen declines, beginning as early as your twenties. Therefore, fine lines, sagging, and loss of elasticity appear. By nourishing collagen production through food and lifestyle, you can slow this process and maintain a firm, radiant complexion longer.

Protein: The Building Blocks of Collagen

Protein provides the amino acids glycine, proline, and hydroxyproline, which are essential for collagen synthesis. Without these building blocks, collagen cannot be formed. This makes daily protein intake one of the most important choices for preserving beauty.

Powerful protein sources include eggs, chicken, fish, beans, lentils, and bone broth. Each of these foods supplies amino acids that feed the body's ability to repair and strengthen skin.

Luxury Tip: A daily serving of bone broth is considered a timeless beauty ritual. Served warm in an elegant cup, it feels both indulgent and restorative, nourishing collagen from within.

The Role of Vitamin C in Collagen Production

Protein provides the raw materials, but Vitamin C is the activator. Without Vitamin C, collagen cannot be formed. Therefore, pairing protein-rich meals with Vitamin C foods is essential.

- Eggs with sautéed spinach.
- Salmon with a side of roasted peppers.
- Grilled chicken with citrus salad.

These combinations transform ordinary meals into collagen-boosting feasts.

Collagen Supplements and Whole Foods

These supplements are beneficial when used with a proper diet. However, whole foods remain the most powerful source of collagen-building nutrients. Bone broth, slow-cooked meats, and plant-based proteins offer amino acids in their most natural and bioavailable form.

Supplements may enhance results, but they should never replace the foundation of real, nutrient-rich meals.

Collagen, Protein, and Aging

As collagen levels decline, the skin becomes thinner and weaker. Yet, women who maintain high-protein diets paired with collagen-boosting foods often show fewer wrinkles and more firmness than those who neglect protein. Aging with elegance is not about avoiding time; it is about nourishing the body so that time enhances rather than diminishes your beauty.

Luxury Rituals for Collagen and Protein Power

Collagen care can become part of your lifestyle in refined ways.

- Begin your morning with a smoothie made of Greek yogurt, berries, and chia seeds.
- Enjoy lunch of quinoa and lentil salad topped with eggs.
- Prepare dinner with grilled fish or roasted chicken paired with colorful vegetables.
- End the evening with a small serving of warm bone broth to support overnight repair.

These rituals do more than feed your body. They create a sense of elegance and intention that transforms eating into beauty care.

Case Study: Firmness Preserved vs. Firmness Lost

Two women in their fifties had similar lifestyles, yet their diets were very different. One consumed minimal protein and relied on refined carbohydrates. Her skin sagged early, her lines deepened, and her complexion lacked structure. The other prioritized protein and paired it with foods rich in Vitamin C. Her skin remained firm, smooth, and radiant, reflecting her consistent commitment to nourishment.

The contrast was striking. The difference was not in effort but in choice. One protein's role in collagen is often overlooked. The other treated it as essential.

Key Takeaway

Collagen is the foundation of firmness, and protein is the fuel that creates it. By combining protein-rich foods with Vitamin C, you activate collagen synthesis and preserve youthful structure in your skin. Supplements may enhance, but whole foods remain the most potent source of support. With daily collagen rituals, you choose a glow that matures with grace, elegance, and strength.

CHAPTER 12

Antioxidants and Superfoods

A radiant complexion is more than skin deep. Every day, your skin faces invisible attackers such as pollution, stress, ultraviolet rays, and poor diet choices. These factors create free radicals, unstable molecules that damage skin cells, accelerate aging, and weaken your glow. The most potent defense against these threats is found in antioxidants.

Antioxidants are nature's anti-aging guardians. They neutralize free radicals, protect collagen, and maintain the skin's vibrancy and strength. Superfoods, which are rich in antioxidants, provide an elegant way to nourish your body with beauty-enhancing protection. With daily rituals that include these foods, you not only slow aging but also cultivate a glow that radiates confidence and vitality.

Why Antioxidants are Anti-Aging

The process of oxidation is inevitable. It occurs when your skin is exposed to sunlight, stress, toxins, or when your body breaks down energy-rich food. Oxidation creates free radicals that damage cells and speed up the visible signs of aging, such as fine lines, dullness, and uneven tone.

Antioxidants step in to restore balance. They neutralize free radicals before harm is done, preserve collagen, and keep your complexion youthful. Therefore, individuals with antioxidant-rich diets often appear younger, with skin that looks more resilient and luminous.

Superfoods that Deliver Radiance

Superfoods are foods packed with extraordinary amounts of antioxidants, vitamins, and minerals. Including them daily transforms meals into beauty treatments.

- Blueberries provide anthocyanins, which fight cellular damage and brighten the complexion.
- Pomegranates protect collagen and reduce inflammation, leaving skin firmer.
- Green tea offers catechins, which protect against UV damage and calm redness.
- Turmeric contains curcumin, known for its powerful anti-inflammatory and brightening effects.
- Dark chocolate delivers flavonoids that increase circulation and hydration in the skin.

Luxury Tip: Curate your pantry with these foods as staples. A simple breakfast of Greek yogurt topped with blueberries and pomegranate seeds becomes an indulgent beauty ritual.

Daily Rituals with Antioxidants

Consistency turns antioxidants into visible radiance. Occasional superfoods are helpful, but daily rituals deliver transformation.

- Begin your day with green tea instead of coffee for a calm yet energized glow.
- Add a teaspoon of turmeric into soups or golden milk for an elegant evening ritual.
- End a meal with a square of dark chocolate, paired with berries for both indulgence and nourishment.
- Incorporate pomegranate seeds into salads or smoothies for a burst of beauty-enhancing nutrients.

These habits feel luxurious while repairing and protecting your skin.

The Antioxidant-Collagen Connection

Antioxidants not only fight free radicals but also protect and stimulate collagen production. This means fewer wrinkles, a stronger skin structure, and longer-lasting firmness. Pairing antioxidants with collagen-supportive foods such as protein and Vitamin C creates a powerful synergy, ensuring your skin ages and keeps its natural elasticity.

Antioxidants and Inflammation

Beyond aging, inflammation is one of the greatest enemies of radiant skin. It causes redness, puffiness, and uneven tone. Antioxidants calm this response, helping the skin appear more even, soothed, and luminous. For individuals prone to acne or irritation, antioxidant-rich diets often reduce flare-ups and create a calmer, more balanced complexion.

Luxury Living with Superfoods

Adding superfoods does not need to feel clinical. It can become a refined lifestyle. Imagine hosting a dinner where guests are served a fresh pomegranate salad, sipping antioxidant-rich green tea in a porcelain cup during the afternoon, or ending an evening with a small piece of artisan dark chocolate. These practices combine elegance with purpose, making beauty a natural outcome of luxurious living.

Case Study: Aging Slowed by Antioxidants

Two women entered their fifties with similar genetics. One consumed a diet heavy in processed foods and relied only on topical creams. Her skin showed signs of early sagging, fine lines, and uneven pigmentation. The other made antioxidants and superfoods part of her daily lifestyle, from green tea in the morning to blueberries at breakfast and dark chocolate after dinner. Her skin appeared firmer, more luminous, and years younger than her age.

The contrast revealed that while creams polish, antioxidants protect and preserve beauty at the deepest level.

Key Takeaway

Antioxidants are your skin's timeless protectors. They neutralize free radicals, preserve collagen, calm inflammation, and slow the visible signs of aging. Superfoods are the most elegant way to deliver these benefits daily, transforming ordinary meals into rituals of radiance. By making antioxidants a consistent part of your lifestyle, you do not just slow aging; you redefine it, choosing beauty that matures with strength and confidence.

Chapter 13

30-Day Food Glow Challenge

Radiance is not built in a single day, and glow is not the result of one meal. True transformation comes from consistency. Therefore, I created the 30-Day Food Glow Challenge, a step-by-step plan designed to guide you toward visible improvements in just one month. Each week introduces new layers of nourishment so your skin receives a steady flow of hydration, vitamins, minerals, and antioxidants. By the end of thirty days, you will not only notice a change in your complexion but also in your energy, your mood, and your confidence.

Think of this challenge as your personal glow retreat at home. Every day, please make intentional, elevated choices that serve your long-term beauty and well-being.

How to Approach the Challenge

This is not a diet. It is a lifestyle upgrade. Each week builds upon the last, creating habits you can carry forward long after the thirty days are complete. The goal is not perfection but consistency. If you miss a meal or slip for a day, continue the next day. Every choice in this challenge is an investment in your glow.

Luxury Tip: Keep a journal or planned for your Glow Challenge. Each day, write the foods you added, how your skin feels, and any changes you notice. Treat it like a beauty diary, a record of your journey toward radiance.

Week 1: Hydration and Vitamin C Foundation

The first week sets the stage by flooding your body with hydration and antioxidants.

- Drink at least half your body weight in ounces of water daily, adding lemon or cucumber for elegance and detox support.
- Begin every morning with warm lemon water or citrus-infused tea.
- Add at least one Vitamin C food to every meal, such as oranges, peppers, strawberries, or kiwi.

By the end of the week, your skin will already feel more hydrated, fresh, and awake.

Week 2: Renewal with Vitamin A and Healthy Fats

In the second week, you begin to strengthen and renew. Vitamin A fuels cell turnover, while healthy fats lock in moisture.

- Add a serving of Vitamin A-rich food daily, such as sweet potatoes, carrots, or spinach.
- Pair these with healthy fats like avocado, olive oil, or nuts to ensure absorption.
- Enjoy at least two servings of omega-3-rich foods, such as salmon, chia seeds, or walnuts.

This week brings a smoother texture, reduced dryness, and the beginning of natural luminosity.

Week 3: Balance with Probiotics and Minerals

By the third week, it is time to support deeper balance through gut health and essential minerals.

- Add one probiotic food daily, such as yogurt, kefir, kimchi, or kombucha.
- Support probiotics with prebiotics such as bananas, onions, garlic, or oats.
- Focus on zinc, selenium, and iron by adding foods like pumpkin seeds, Brazil nuts, spinach, or lentils.

This stage calms inflammation, supports even tone, and builds a firm foundation for long-term radiance.

Week 4: Antioxidant Superfoods and Collagen Support

The last week elevates your glow to its fullest by layering in collagen support and high-antioxidant superfoods.

- Include a collagen-supportive protein daily, such as chicken, fish, beans, or bone broth. Pair it with Vitamin C foods to activate collagen production.
- Choose at least one superfood daily, such as blueberries, pomegranates, turmeric, green tea, or dark chocolate.
- Continue hydration rituals and probiotic support to reinforce your foundation.

This week helps skin look firmer, brighter, and more refined, creating a radiance that lasts far beyond the thirty days.

Integrating Lifestyle with Nutrition

The challenge is not only about food but about rituals. Elevate your meals into experiences. Drink water from a beautiful glass, serve colorful salads on elegant plates, and take a mindful pause while enjoying antioxidant-rich tea. By treating each step as a luxury act of self-care, you transform the challenge into a celebration.

Case Study: Thirty Days to Transformation

One client approached this challenge with tired skin, frequent breakouts, and low energy. She followed each week with consistency, keeping a glow journal as recommended. Within ten days, she noticed her skin was less dry. By the second week, her breakouts calmed. In week three, her under-eye circles faded, and by the end of thirty days, her skin tone was brighter and more even. Beyond her appearance, she reported more energy, an improved mood, and a renewed sense of confidence.

Her transformation was not luck but a reflection of daily choices.

Key Takeaway

The 30-Day Food Glow Challenge is your invitation to reset, renew, and reveal your radiance. By layering hydration, vitamins, minerals, probiotics, antioxidants, and collagen support, you create a glow plan that transforms not only your skin but your lifestyle. Thirty days is just the beginning. These habits are the foundation of a beauty legacy that can last a lifetime.

CHAPTER 14

Recipes for Radiance

Glowing skin is not only built in the kitchen but also experienced at the table. Food is more than nourishment; it is a ritual, a moment of beauty that begins with intention and ends with radiance. These recipes deliver nutrients that strengthen collagen, calm inflammation, and flood your body with antioxidants. They're straightforward enough for everyday use, but still feel special.

The Glow Smoothie

A morning ritual that feels like a spa treatment in a glass. This blend hydrates, energies, and prepares your skin for the day ahead.

Ingredients:

- Spinach for chlorophyll and iron, which oxygenates the skin.

- Pineapple for Vitamin C and natural enzymes that brighten tone.
- Chia seeds for omega-3 fatty acids that moisturize from within.
- Lemon water for hydration and detoxification.

Luxury Ritual: Serve in a tall glass with a slice of lemon on the rim. Drink, allowing each sip to feel like a renewal.

The Skin-Repair Salad

This salad rebuilds and restore. It is packed with vitamins, minerals, and healthy fats that help repair the skin barrier and maintain a resilient glow.

Ingredients:

- Kale for Vitamin K, which supports circulation and balance.
- Avocado for nourishing fats that lock in moisture.
- Pumpkin seeds for zinc, which calms acne and supports healing.
- Olive oil for Vitamin E, which shields and protects.

Luxury Ritual: Toss and serve on a white plate to let the vibrant green colors shine. Add a squeeze of lemon for brightness.

The Omega Bowl

A meal that delivers strength and suppleness. The Omega Bowl helps fuel collagen, preserves elasticity, and leaves the skin more luminous.

Ingredients:

- Salmon for omega-3s, which reduce inflammation and moisturize.
- Quinoa for protein to support collagen production.
- Sweet potatoes for beta-carotene, which renews and smooths.
- Leafy greens for minerals that strengthen and protect.

Luxury Ritual: Arrange each component in the bowl, creating a palette of colors. Drizzle with olive oil to elevate both flavor and glow.

The Gut-Healing Soup

Calm, restorative, and nourishing, this soup supports digestion, balances the microbiome, and soothes the skin from the inside out.

Ingredients:

- Bone broth for collagen and minerals that repair tissue.
- Garlic for prebiotic fibers that fuel healthy bacteria.
- Mushrooms for antioxidants and immune support.

- Turmeric for anti-inflammatory benefits and radiance.

Luxury Ritual: Serve in a ceramic bowl with a sprig of parsley on top. Sip in the evening to prepare the body and skin for overnight renewal.

The Chocolate Glow Bites

A sweet indulgence that proves radiant living can also be decadent. These bites satisfy cravings while feeding your skin with antioxidants and healthy fats.

Ingredients:

- Dark chocolate for flavonoids that improve circulation and hydration.
- Walnuts for omega-3s and protein to strengthen collagen.
- Cranberries for Vitamin C and antioxidants to brighten.

Luxury Ritual: Place on a small plate, paired with a cup of green tea for balance. Enjoy, knowing every bite is both indulgence and nourishment.

Bringing Recipes for Daily Life

These recipes are more than instructions. They are designed as rituals of beauty. By preparing them with intention and serving them with elegance, you turn ordinary meals into experiences that reflect the lifestyle of radiance you are building. Consistency transforms these recipes from occasional treats into the foundation of your glow.

Key Takeaway

Food is your most powerful beauty treatment. By incorporating these nutrient-rich recipes into your daily rhythm, you create a lifestyle where every meal strengthens your skin, enhances your glow, and reminds you that self-care can be both simple and luxurious.

Chapter 15

Troubleshooting Skin Through Food

Even with the best routines, skin sometimes reveals signs of imbalance. Acne, dryness, dark circles, and dullness are not random problems but messages from the body. Instead of masking them with makeup or quick fixes, the most powerful approach is to address their root causes through nutrition. Food has the power to rebalance, restore, and renew your skin.

This chapter is your guide to identifying common skin concerns and using targeted nourishment as your solution. Each change becomes not only a treatment but also a long-term investment in radiant health.

Acne: Calm the Inflammation, Restore the Balance

Acne often begins with internal inflammation, excess oil, and imbalanced hormones. Processed sugar and dairy products are two of the strongest dietary triggers, as they increase insulin levels and stimulate oil production.

By reducing or eliminating these triggers, the body calms inflammation. Nourishing the skin with healing foods strengthens its ability to fight breakouts.

- Add zinc-rich foods such as pumpkin seeds, oysters, and lentils to regulate oil and speed healing.
- Incorporate probiotic foods such as yogurt, kefir, and kimchi to balance the gut, reducing inflammation that contributes to acne.
- Drink plenty of water to flush toxins and keep skin clear.

Luxury Ritual: Replace sugary snacks with a small bowl of Greek yogurt topped with pumpkin seeds and fresh berries. It feels indulgent, supports gut balance, and provides nutrients that calm the skin from within.

Dryness: Nourish with Moisture from Within

Dry skin is often a signal that the body lacks healthy fats or hydration. While creams can soothe the surface, true transformation begins with what you consume.

- Include omega-3-rich foods such as salmon, chia seeds, flaxseeds, and walnuts to provide lasting hydration.
- Drink water throughout the day, pairing it with electrolytes from fruits and coconut water to improve absorption.

- Add hydrating fruits and vegetables such as cucumbers, watermelon, and oranges to support water retention in the skin.

Luxury Ritual: Begin the day with a chia seed pudding topped with slices of kiwi and a drizzle of almond milk. It hydrates, nourishes, and delivers glow-enhancing omega-3s in a refined way.

Dark Circles: Strengthen and Brighten from the Inside

Dark circles are not only the result of lack of sleep. They can also be caused by weak capillaries, poor circulation, or nutrient deficiencies. Vitamin K and iron are two of the most effective nutrients for restoring brightness under the eyes.

- Eat Vitamin K-rich greens such as spinach, kale, and parsley to strengthen capillaries and reduce shadowing.
- Add iron-rich foods such as lentils, spinach, and lean meats to improve oxygen delivery and brighten skin tone.
- Pair iron with Vitamin C foods such as citrus or peppers to enhance absorption.

Luxury Ritual: Prepare a vibrant spinach salad with roasted peppers and a sprinkle of fresh parsley. Not only is it elegant, but it also delivers a concentrated dose of Vitamin K and iron.

Dullness: Restore Light with Antioxidants and Vitamin C

Dull skin often shows a lack of antioxidants and Vitamin C. Without these nutrients, free radicals accumulate, damaging cells and leaving skin lifeless. By replenishing antioxidants, you restore vitality and brightness.

- Add Vitamin C-rich foods such as oranges, kiwi, strawberries, and bell peppers to stimulate collagen and illuminate the complexion.
- Choose antioxidant superfoods such as blueberries, pomegranates, green tea, and dark chocolate to defend against oxidative stress.
- Ensure that every meal includes at least one colorful fruit or vegetable to keep skin nourished.

Luxury Ritual: Replace your afternoon coffee with a cup of green tea, paired with a square of dark chocolate and a handful of blueberries. It feels indulgent, energizing the body and reviving the glow of your skin.

Case Study: Skin Renewed Through Food

One woman in her thirties struggled with multiple concerns: breakouts, dryness, and dark circles. She had tried countless creams without lasting results. Once she began adjusting her diet, reducing sugar and dairy while adding probiotics, greens, omega-3s, and antioxidants, her skin transformed. Breakouts subsided, hydration returned, and her under-eye area appeared brighter. Her friends quickly became curious about her skincare routine, although the solution was straightforward: nutrition as a remedy.

Key Takeaway

Your skin concerns are not permanent problems. They are signals from the body that can be answered with nourishment. Acne, dryness, dark circles, and dullness can all be addressed through targeted foods that heal from the inside out. By choosing nutrition as your primary troubleshooting tool, you empower yourself to create lasting radiance without relying on temporary fixes.

Chapter 16

Building Your Long-Term Glow Plan

A thirty-day glow challenge is potent, but everlasting radiance requires a lifetime of work. The realistic goal is not temporary results but a lifestyle that sustains your beauty for years. Glow is not a destination; it is a rhythm, a daily set of choices that become second nature. When food, hydration, and mindful rituals become part of your lifestyle, your skin no longer reflects the need for quick fixes. It reflects legacy.

This chapter serves as your guide to transforming everything you have learned into a comprehensive long-term plan. It is about creating habits that are effortless, enjoyable, and aligned with your vision of elegance and vitality.

The Power of Consistency

Skin thrives on routine. Just as topical care requires a daily commitment, so does food care. It is not the occasional salad or smoothie that changes your skin, but the choices you make every day.

- Consistency with hydration ensures plumpness and resilience.
- Consistency with vitamins and minerals ensures steady renewal.
- Consistency with probiotics ensures a lasting balance in the gut-skin connection.

The luxury of glow comes not from effort but from rhythm.

Seasonal Adjustments for Lasting Radiance

Your skin's needs shift with the seasons, and your diet can adapt.

- In summer, emphasize hydration, light fruits, and cooling vegetables such as cucumber and watermelon.
- In winter, focus on warming soups, bone broth, and omega-rich foods that lock in moisture.
- In spring, embrace detoxifying greens to renew after the heavier months.
- In the fall, choose antioxidant-rich foods such as pomegranates, squash, and dark leafy greens.

By aligning nutrition with the seasons, your skin receives what it needs to thrive year-round.

Lifestyle Integration: Turning Habits Into Rituals

The key to maintaining radiance is to elevate simple habits into refined rituals. When wellness feels indulgent, consistency is effortless.

- Hydration becomes more enjoyable when served in a crystal glass or infused with citrus.
- Eating greens feels elegant when arranged on a plate with care.
- Preparing bone broth in the evening becomes a calming ritual rather than a task.

The more you connect beauty care to luxury living, the more sustainable it becomes.

Balancing Indulgence and Discipline

A sustainable glow plan does not demand perfection. There is space for indulgence, as long as balance is maintained. Enjoy the occasional dessert or celebratory meal, knowing that your foundation of nourishment will keep your skin resilient and healthy. Discipline ensures structure, while indulgence ensures joy. Together, they create a balanced approach that lasts.

The Role of Mindset in Long-Term Radiance

True glow begins in the mind. When you believe that every choice is an investment in your beauty and health, you eat, drink, and live with intention. This mindset transforms ordinary decisions into influential acts of self-care.

Instead of thinking, "I must eat healthy," think, "I choose radiance." This shift transforms discipline into empowerment, making your glow plan something you look forward to rather than something you endure.

Legacy of Radiance

What makes Glow sustainable is not only how it looks but how it feels. Radiance is energy, confidence, and the grace with which you carry yourself. When you incorporate your glow plan into your daily life, you create a legacy of wellness that everyone around you will notice. People will not just see your skin; they will see your vitality, your strength, and your elegance.

Case Study: The Woman Who Chose Longevity

One woman in her forties embraced the thirty-day glow challenge and then transitioned into a long-term lifestyle. She continued her hydration rituals, adjusted her meals according to the seasons, and treated food as beauty care. Ten years later, she was often mistaken for being younger than she was. Her friends admired not only her complexion but also her energy and grace.

Her secret was not expensive treatments. It was consistency, refinement, and intention.

Key Takeaway

Glow is not a short-term result but a long-term lifestyle. By embracing consistency, adjusting with the seasons, transforming habits into rituals, and balancing discipline with indulgence, you create a beauty plan that endures. Your glow becomes part of your identity, a legacy of health and elegance that grows stronger with time.

Conclusion

Your Glow Journey

Radiance is never the result of chance. It is the outcome of consistent, intentional choices that honor your body every single day. Throughout this book, you have learned how hydration, vitamins, minerals, probiotics, antioxidants, and proteins all work together to create beauty from within. These are not temporary solutions but timeless foundations.

The 30-Day Glow Challenge provided a starting structure, but true transformation occurs when you continue these practices as a lifestyle. Glow is not a quick fix or a passing trend. It is a rhythm—a way of eating, living, and caring for yourself that becomes second nature. Every colorful plate, every sip of water, every probiotic meal is a quiet act of self-respect and self-investment.

Your glow will always reflect more than skin. It will be evident in your energy, confidence, and the presence you bring to every room. When people notice your radiance, they will not only see beauty but also your inner light. They will sense the care, discipline, and grace behind it.

Embrace your glow as part of who you are. Protect it with nourishing choices, elevate it with daily rituals, and carry it as your signature. This is not only about looking luminous today—it is about building a legacy of beauty, health, and vitality that matures with you.

About the Author

Stephanie Williams, MBA — Strategic Business Consultant, author, and builder of beauty, brains, and business.

Stephanie is a visionary entrepreneur, and publishing powerhouse who helps others shine from the inside out. With an MBA from the Jack Welch Management Institute (perfect GPA, with a concentration in entrepreneurship) and years of experience at Verizon and Verizon Connect, she has developed expertise in corporate strategy and sales before building her own brand.

Her personal journey inspired her to write Blow Up Skincare and the 30-Day Food-Based Skin Health Book, uniting topical care with food-based strategies. Through Booked & Branded Publishing, she helps clients transform ideas into polished, profitable books and digital products.

When she isn't building brands and books, Stephanie curates wellness routines, empowers entrepreneurs, and designs a life where hustle meets strategy.

Work With Me

Your credit journey doesn't have to end here.
If this book spoke to you and you're ready to go deeper, there are ways we can walk this path together:

1:1 Consulting & Strategic Guidance

Personalized sessions designed to help you uncover blind spots, create actionable strategies, and reach your financial goals.

Workshops, Masterclasses & Keynotes

From group coaching to private training, I equip individuals and organizations with practical tools for building strong credit and financial empowerment.

Booked and Branded Publishing™

If you've ever dreamed of writing a book of your own, I can guide you through the process — from clarifying your message, to building your brand, to publishing with excellence.

Let's Connect

Website:https://www.bookedandbrandedpublishing.com/
Email: hello@bookedandbrandedpublishing.com

Don't let this book end on the page.
Let it live in your life. Let's build something extraordinary — together.

Thank you for reading. We've included a free downloadable workbook to help you apply these principles.

Scan for FREE WORKBOOK Printable Tracker & Digital Copy

Acknowledgments

To my family and friends who reminded me that even when I wanted to hide, I was seen — thank you. To my clients and community, who have trusted me with their journeys, thank you for proving that growth is not just possible — it's contagious. And to you, the reader: thank you for your courage. You are proof that it is possible to live and unmasked.

Stephanie Williams, MBA — Strategic Business Consultant, author, and builder of beauty, brains, and business.

Thank you for your purchase! I'd appreciate it if you could write a short Amazon review, assuming this book has been helpful. Your words help others find this message and remind them they are not alone.

Scan QR Code to leave a Review

Made in the USA
Monee, IL
12 November 2026

92be0bbd-38e0-4def-b250-8f7c663ef768R01